Whole Foods: Could It Be Your Secret to Losing Weight?

Lose Weight Eating Bounty From Mother Earth

RON KNESS

Contents

Disclaimer

This publication is for informational purposes only and is not intended as medical advice. Medical advice should always be obtained from a qualified medical professional for any health conditions or symptoms associated with them.

Every possible effort has been made in preparing and researching this material. We make no warranties with respect to the accuracy, applicability of its contents or any omissions.

See your healthcare professional before starting any diet or exercise program!

Introduction

Weight loss ... it is something that millions of Americans struggle with. Every year millions of dollars are poured into the dieting and fitness market in hopes that something will finally be the breakthrough to weight loss success. But the truth is these diet trends make losing weight seem much harder than it needs to be, and even worse many times these diets are not a healthy way to lose weight. Sure, you may drop some pounds, you may even keep it off for a while ... but that doesn't always mean that the things you are eating are not doing damage to your body. Contrary to popular belief it is very possible to lose weight without the method you are using being healthy.

What you need to truly lose weight isn't the next diet gimmick or a multitude of supplements. You don't need those perfectly portioned frozen foods, and you don't need to count calories or starve yourself waiting for your next scheduled meal time. All of this stuff makes losing weight much more complicated than it needs to be.

And the biggest fault with most diets is they are not sustainable. Most of them are so rigid that you can't stay on them forever and when you do come off, you gain back the weight you lost and in most cases, more. In the end, you weight more now than when you first started your diet.

Losing weight can be simple, it can be easy, and it can be effortless. Weight loss isn't about making things more complicated, it is actually about simplifying your life.

When you learn how to live off of foods in their most natural state – whole foods - you will see a transformation in your body. Not only will your body be able to naturally flush out anything that it doesn't need, but it will also be able to absorb nutrients much faster and even cure many of your health issues.

This is why so many people find themselves turning to whole foods. When you are eating whole foods, you are eating foods that are going to give your body everything that it needs to be truly healthy. You are also giving your body the foods that it was naturally designed to eat.

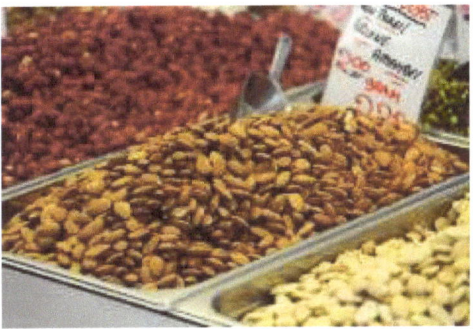

Think about it, many of the foods in the average diet are things that were made by man, not by nature. And these foods are typically loaded with things that our bodies simply cannot digest, leaving us fat, unhealthy, and prone to developing sicknesses or even cancer.

Sugars, dyes, and processed foods are just a few examples of the things that can wreak havoc on our digestive system. Because your body was not made to eat these things, it has to work extra hard to push them through the system, and whatever it cannot get through your system will turn into unwanted fat and extra weight.

Whole foods aren't like that though. When you eat whole foods, your body can quickly take that food, digest it, and move it through your system.

Because your body won't be bogged down with digestion, it will have time to start cleaning out unwanted things that are trapped in your system, (typically fat cells). this is how people who are on a whole foods diet able to lose weight quickly.

In addition, people find that they have more energy, sleep better, and return to their natural weight faster than they ever thought possible.

To Your Success!

List Your Whole Foods Goal

Whether you are trying to lose weight with whole foods or you have another eating path that you are taking, it is always important to have goals before you start any eating or weight loss journey. Goals will give you something to strive for, and they will help you to find motivation during those times when you might otherwise feel like giving up. Losing weight can be hard, and there will be times when you will struggle. This struggle can be dangerous as it can sabotage your ability to successfully lose the weight, or keep it off.

But when you have goals set in place, you have something that

will get you through any potential stumbling blocks in your weight loss journey. Goals will provide that motivation you need when things get tough, and they will help you to push through any barriers you will face along the way.

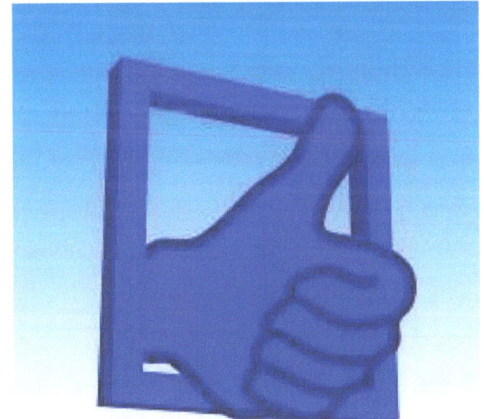

When it comes to making goals, it isn't a question of whether or not they will help you in your weight loss journey, it is a question of how you should best put your goals into place. The following are a few simple tips that will help you to not only create goals, but create goals that will help you find success in the fastest way possible.

Start Small

It might be a bit frustrating at first, but when it comes to goals you want to start by starting small. To be successful, goals have to be realistic and attainable. If your goals are too far reaching, it will make them seem impossible to achieve during those times when things get rough …. and they will get rough! On the other hand, if your goals seem reachable, then it will be much easier for you to find your motivation when you need it most. The reason is because that goal will seem just within your reach.

Yes, you likely have big goals that you want to achieve and yes, you will be able to achieve them. But when we look at the end result, we sometimes lose focus of the smaller steps it takes to get there.

Let's think about it in a different way, let's look at a successful business like Whole Foods. When someone set out to create the first Whole Foods Market, do you think they had nothing but the big picture in mind? Do you think their only mission was to create a large chain of Whole Food stores that would serve fresh, natural, healthy foods? Or do you think that they broke that 'big goal' down into smaller goals that shifted over time?

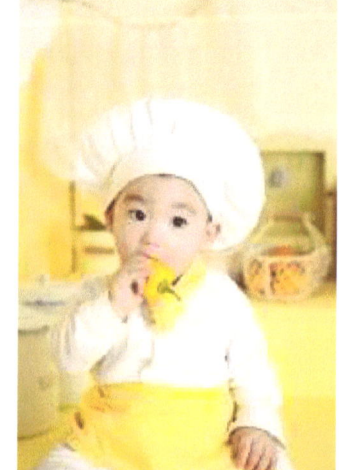

Your weight loss journey is no different. When you are preparing to lose weight, you don't just want to look at the end result, you also want to look at the smaller steps you will need to take to get there.

When you approach weight loss this way you aren't just setting yourself up for immediate success, you are also setting yourself up for ongoing success in the future.

Reward Yourself

Another thing that you can do to stay focused on your weight loss journey is to plan rewards for yourself. Rewarding yourself serves two main purposes.

First, it allows you to feel good about yourself. This is important because there will be parts of your weight loss journey where you might be feeling under the weather and that might break you down a bit emotionally.

But when you reward yourself, you are practicing a bit of self-love and you are giving yourself a bit of praise for the job that you have done.

Second, rewarding yourself allows you to keep your motivation throughout your weight loss journey. There are going to be times when things get hard. There will be times when you want to quit and you are tempted to fall off of your new eating path.

Things like dining out with friends, having a bad day at work, and celebrating special occasions are all things that can be linked to your old eating habits, and when these things occur, it might be a bit challenging to stay focused on your weight loss success.

But if you are always inches away from accomplishing your next healthy eating goal, then it will be much easier for you to avoid these temptations because you will be so excited about cashing in on your next reward.

Your rewards don't have to be lavish and they definitely shouldn't be linked to the unhealthy foods that you are trying to get away from. Instead, your rewards should be something that makes you happy and makes you feel like you are treating yourself to something special. Some examples include:

- A trip to the movies

- A beauty product you want but haven't gotten around to getting

- A few new clothes

- A small vacation or trip

Re-Evaluate Often

As you go through your weight loss journey, you will find that your goals begin to shift. This could be because you have started to accomplish these goals and you are ready to move onto the next set of goals. It could also mean that as your journey is evolving, your whole food weight loss goals are evolving as well.

Both of these are good things. They mean that you are progressing, stretching, and growing as a person. They are also the reason why you want to be sure that you are re-evaluating your goals often.

Once one goal has passed, you want to be ready to jump right into the next one, if you wait until a goal is complete before you start thinking about the next one, you will have a period of 'space' where you are not trying to accomplish any goals, but simply coasting on your journey for a bit. This can be a dangerous game when you are trying to achieve something like weight loss.

You never want to have any downtime when it comes to your goals, you always want to be able to know exactly where you have been, where you are, and where you are going.

How often should you be evaluating your goals? That is really a personal decision, but checking in with yourself a few days before you accomplish one goal might be a good idea. If you are in the middle of a huge life change, for example a move, then you might want to evaluate your goals every few days so that you can better handle the stress and changes you are facing. On the other hand if your life is in a stable place and you have been successfully losing weight with little effort, you don't need to check in with your goals as often because they will likely not change much.

Find Your Biggest Obstacle

Now that you have identified your goals, it is time to switch gears and look for your biggest obstacles. These are not meant to be things that hinder you from success. This is not meant to scare you and it definitely isn't meant to make you feel like you can't succeed on this journey.

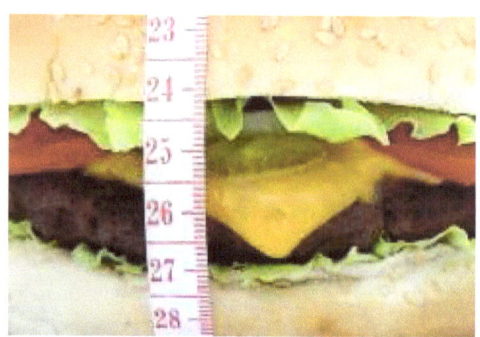

Finding your biggest obstacles is a great way to figure out what your plan will be to get around these obstacles. Once you have a plan in place, you will be prepared when these challenges arise and they will not be able to sidetrack you from your weight loss goals.

When you are thinking about your obstacles, it is a good idea to think about the obstacles that can arise throughout your whole journey, not just the immediate future. Also, don't overlook thinking about obstacles that have prevented you from having success in your weight loss journey in the past. They may still be there. After all, we rarely know what life will throw at us and having a plan in place will help us to be prepared for anything new or old.

Are there any major life events that might be happening? Are there going to be traveling or changing careers or expanding your family in the next year?

All of these things are good things that can be considered obstacles when it comes to weight loss.

Write Them Down

Once you have started to identify your obstacles, it is a good idea to write everything down. This will not only give you a visual record of those obstacles, it will also allow you to have everything in one place when you need it. Most importantly, writing down your obstacles will allow you to write down the solutions to those obstacles as well.

For example, let's say that you are planning on moving within the next year. This is definitely a blessing for you, but it can be an obstacle when it comes to losing weight. You may be moving away from that all-organic market that you love, or your mortgage payment might be increasing. These are the types of things that can put a lot of emotional stress on a person, and potentially cause you to go back to old eating patterns.

But when you have already thought of a solution to that problem, and you have that solution in a place where you can easily reference it, then you will be able to get through that obstacle quickly. What could have easily thrown you off track with your weight loss is now something that you can easily overcome.

Finding Your Mindset

One of the biggest challenges that many people face when they are starting on a new life path is mindset. Yes, the physical decisions that you make on your weight loss journey, or any journey for that matter, are important. But the emotional aspect of your journey is important as well, and make no mistake, if you are not in the correct mindset when you start taking your journey, it will be almost impossible for you to succeed. Losing weight is as much of a mental journey as it is physical. If you are not all in when you start, you will not be successful. In my book *Set Your Mind and The Body Will Follow*, I talk about how important mindset is and some ways to change your mindset.

And you have to want to lose weight. This may sound strange because why would you be on a weight-loss journey if you didn't want to lose weight. It happens all the time. You may be going through the motions of losing weight because someone else in your life wanted you to. Until it becomes your idea, you will not be successful. Being in the right mindset at the start of your journey is paramount to success.

Forgive the Past

One of the most important parts of having a healthy mindset is forgiving yourself for the past. Because the past is just that, the past. It doesn't matter what you have done before today, it doesn't even matter what you have done this morning, all that matters is what you are doing now, and what you are going to do from this point forward.

When you don't forgive yourself for your past relationship with food, you will automatically add a bit of stress to yourself when you begin trying to lose weight. You will have more pressure on yourself to succeed because you will be remembering those times when you were not successful.

Even more important, you might find you are a bit resentful of those healthy eating goals that you were not able to meet in the past, and that resentment can greatly affect your self-esteem and motivation today and even prevent you from being successful. Don't sabotage yourself before you even begin! You can't change the past, so why dwell on it.

However you can learn from it and not repeat bad habits.

Speak to Yourself Kindly

The way that we speak to ourselves has a lasting impact on the

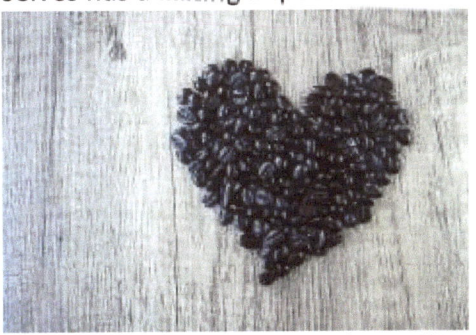

way that we see ourselves and this impact could be a good thing or a bad thing. For those who know how to speak to themselves kindly and with love, they find that their weight loss challenges are more easy to overcome, mainly because they will be able to approach the situation calmly.

On the other hand, people who tend to speak to themselves negatively often find that they have a much harder time dealing with any challenges they face when trying to lose weight.

Typically when they hit an obstacle in their weight loss they become overcome with frustration and fear, and many times this causes them to throw their hands up and walk away from their weight loss journey all together.

Visualize Often

Have you ever heard of the power of visualization? Essentially it is when you are able to create an image in your mind of what you want to accomplish, and then you will hold onto that image until it becomes a reality. When you are trying to lose weight, visualization can be critical for success.

How To Do It

Create a picture in your mind of what you want to accomplish with your weight loss goals. Be very detailed and specific about every aspect of what you want. This one simple trick can have you hitting your goal weight in no time.

Remember, when it comes to losing weight your action are only part of the equation. Without having the proper mindset for success you could very well be setting yourself up for failure.

I delve into the topic of mindset deeper in my book **Change Your Dieting Mindset And Keep That Weight Off Forever!**

Determine Your Eating Path

Making the choice to eat whole foods to lose weight is going to do amazing things for your body, your mind, and your overall health. Whole foods are delicious and they are filled of the crucial nutrients that our bodies crave.

But making the decision to eat whole foods can also be a tricky one. Believe it or not, there are many people who believe themselves to be whole food eaters, and yet they don't always follow the whole food path.

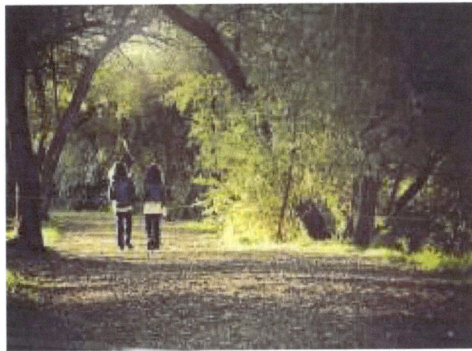

Unlike deciding to be vegetarian or vegan, eating whole foods seems to offer a bit of an unusual variety. And while this is good, you are eating foods fresh from the earth after all, it can also be tricky to someone new to whole foods if they don't properly understand their choices.

Whole Food Eaters

Most people who choose to eat whole foods are just considered 'people who eat whole foods', they don't have any other title than that. These folks typically follow Whole30 or paleo-type approach to eating whole.

They don't typically eat grains, although some do, and they are allowed to eat meat. Typically, they will also avoid:

- Dairy

- Processed Foods

- Sugars

- Gluten

When eating this way, the aim is to primarily eat organic fruits, vegetables, and meat.

Whole Food Vegan/Whole Food Plant Based

There is another form of whole food eaters, and they typically refer to themselves as a 'whole food vegan' or a 'whole food plant based'. These folks do not eat meat, obviously, but will usually find their protein in grains. It is important to note that some whole food plant based eaters *don't* choose to eat grains. But for those that do, they typically follow a 'Forks Over Knives' approach to eating whole.

Typically, whole food vegans and whole food plant based eaters will also avoid:

- Dairy

- Processed Foods

- Sugars

- Gluten

- Oils

Although both of these eating paths are different, they both rely heavily on eating foods in their most natural state.

Perhaps one of the reasons that so many people opt to follow the whole foods eating path is because there is no 'right ' or 'wrong' way to approach a whole food journey, it is what works best for you and your needs. I cover a type of paleo diet in my book **The Plant-Based Paleo Diet Guide.**

How Whole Foods Can Help You Lose Weight

When it comes to eating healthy, choosing the right eating path is hard. There are so many diets and weight loss programs out there that each claim to be best way to lose weight and keep it off. It can be hard to choose the path that is right for you. Add to that the amount of money each of these things costs and the amount of energy and time that is usually required to achieve those weight loss goals and it can be downright overwhelming. And as you may know, that feeling of overwhelm can often lead to your diet failing before it even starts.

But if we are being honest, there is more to this than just weight loss. There is also a health component to consider. Even if a diet helps you to lose weight, it doesn't always mean that it helps you to get healthy. In fact, sometimes it means quite the opposite and can pave the way for health complications later in life.

This is why it is so important to pick an eating plan that is fresh from the earth, something that is pure and natural and made to work with your body instead of working against it. In other words, this is why so many are starting to look to whole foods for their weight loss needs.

Whole foods are unprocessed. This means that they follow your body's natural way of eating. This is important for a few reasons. First, it is easy on the digestive system, which in turn will allow your body to keep all of the energy that it usually loses during digestion, remove waste at a faster speed, and absorb nutrients faster.

When the digestion is slow all of these things, and more, become affected. Many times we don't even realize the amount of energy our bodies have to put into digesting our everyday foods, and most people find themselves pleasantly surprised when they are able to digest foods easily.

Whole foods also encourage the body's natural detoxification process. Let's face it, we simply weren't made to eat a lot of the foods that are part a standard diet. These foods usually contain sugars, processed ingredients, and other things that can be hard on the body. But a diet in whole foods, especially one that is rich in fruits and vegetables, allows the body to focus on cleaning itself out instead of having to work overtime on digestion. When the body detoxifies, it naturally gets rid of waste, cleans pores, freshens breath, and encourages overall weight loss.

Another wonderful gift of eating whole foods is that your body has the chance to be truly nourished. So many of us lack nourishment in our diets, and we don't even know it.

Even if we eat 'healthy', it doesn't necessarily mean that the foods we are eating are actually providing us the correct nourishment. Eating whole tends to mean eating foods that are high in fiber, high in hydration, and high in nourishment, all of which leads to easy weight loss for you.

Losing weight can be a struggle, and for many of us it can seem downright impossible. But when we trust in foods that are whole and unprocessed, we are allowing our bodies to heal from past food choices, while also allowing the body to naturally return itself to its perfect weight.

The Importance of Eating Light to Heavy

Have you ever eaten a 'hearty' meal at breakfast only to go through the rest of the day paying for that decision? Has it ever felt like you just couldn't stay awake, be productive, or just feel good for the rest of the day when you have eaten this way?

It might be a bit hard to admit, but perhaps what we were taught when we were young wasn't the best thing for us. The myth that we couldn't leave the house until we ate something that would 'stick to our ribs' actually did us more harm than good. While 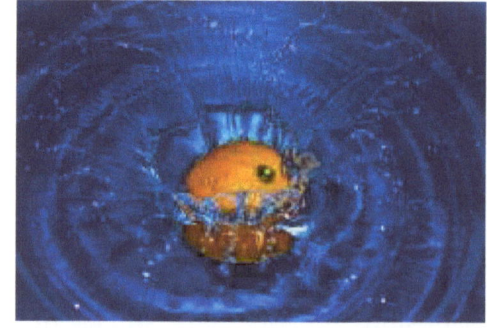 well-meaning parents were trying to do what they believed was best, over time there has been much research that has shown that some of the things that were once considered staples of the American diet might have actually been contributing to our poor health.

Things like eating pancakes for breakfast might actually be the cause for our mid-morning slump. That breakfast sandwich with a glass of milk may have seemed like an easy way to eat while running out of the door, but it may also be responsible for that strange stomach ache that you develop later in the day.

Our bodies were simply not made to eat this way. We were just not designed to wake up and load ourselves up with heavy foods that do not digest easily. This is why it is so important to eat light in the morning to heavy later in the day.

Maintain Energy

Have you ever woken up in the morning and felt like you had gotten a good night's sleep, only to feel like you need coffee by midday? If you are journaling your eating choices and daily habits, you will likely notice there is a pattern between your mid-day slump and your intake for the day.

Here's the thing, when you first wake up in the morning, your body has just spent the entire night digesting your food. Yes, while you are sleeping your body is still working. This is the reason why we tend to feel more energetic during the morning hours.

Eating light to heavy is an easy way to maintain your energy throughout the day because you will not be asking your body to digest heavy foods after it has just spent all night 'cleaning house'.

Speed Up Digestion

In a way, this goes along with maintaining energy. When you eat light to heavy throughout the day, you are giving your digestive system a break.

When the first thing that you eat is processed foods, which are very hard for your body to digest, you will spend the rest of the day digesting that food.

And no matter what you do, you will not be able to reverse the effects of that heavy meal.

For example, let's say that you ate a bagel and cream cheese for breakfast, but you decided that you were going to eat a large salad for lunch and salmon for dinner. On the surface, it would look like you had an overall healthy day. But the reality is that the bagel is making it impossible for your other meals to be digested.

Sure, that salad would normally be something your body would digest quickly, but because your body needs to focus on digesting that bagel, it will digest that salad much more slowly.

Allow Room for You to Slip Up

One of the best gifts that you give yourself when you eat light to heavy is the ability to slip up and recover quickly. When you are staring a whole food weight loss journey, you might find that it is very tempting to eat something that is part of your old diet. If you give into this temptation in the morning hours, it will leave you feeling sluggish, and likely guilty, for the rest of the day.

But if you give in to a craving in the evening, after eating healthy all day, you will find that it is much easier for you to bounce back into your healthy eating routine the next day. This is mainly because your body has the time it needs to work on the hard job of digesting that unhealthy food, and it doesn't have to worry about digesting any other meals after that. This means that you will have little to no ill effects from your food choices.

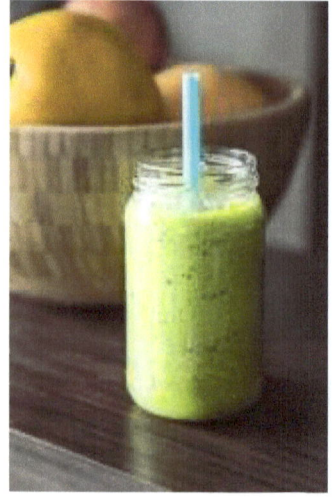

These are just a few of the reasons it is so important to eat light to heavy. When you are able to work with your digestion, you will find that you will not only lose weight more quickly, but you will also have more energy doing it.

What Is Allowed

One of the biggest setbacks when trying to find a new eating path is figuring out what you are allowed to eat. So many times we start a new eating path and quickly become bored or frustrated with our food choices. Worse yet, sometimes we start a new eating path and we aren't sure what we are allowed to eat, so we mistakenly eat the wrong thing, which will hinder us in our weight loss goals. This is why it is important to stick with an eating plan that has foods that you are familiar with, foods that you know your body is used to eating, and most importantly foods that offer an abundance of health.

This is why so many people turn to whole foods. When you are eating whole foods, it is pretty easy to determine what you can

and cannot eat. It's all very straightforward with little room for error. For starters, you know that you are looking for unprocessed foods and foods that the body is able to digest easily. If it doesn't 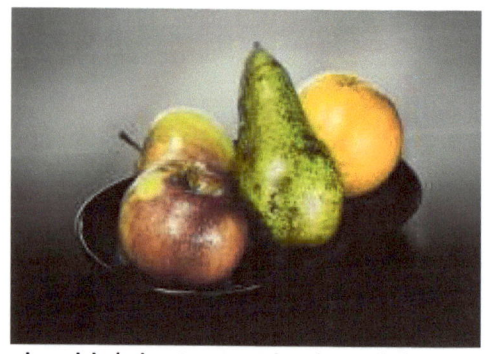 come from the earth, it likely shouldn't be in your body. While many whole food eaters choose to eat meat, the aim is to eat organic meat as that meat source should have been on a diet of foods that came from the earth.

You also want to stick with organic foods. Because these are free of harmful chemicals, they provide the body with more nutrients than non-organic foods.

While eating organic can seem intimidating at first , mainly due to its higher price, it is a true investment in your health. Over time, people who eat organic tend to get sick less and need medication less, making the higher price of organic food well worth it.

These are just a few of the things you can eat on a whole food plan. If you are still unsure which foods you are able to eat on a whole food diet, you can always check the Whole30.com website. This is where you will get a list of recommended whole foods as well as in-depth descriptions about the foods that you want to eat and why those foods are important. Many people are happily surprised to learn that they can still eat many of the foods that they are familiar with.

As a final thought, it is important to remember that eating whole does not mean that you are never allowed to eat processed foods again. Almost every diet allows you to have 'cheats' so that you don't get burned out. Eating whole is no different. Yes, in a perfect world you would eat whole all of the time, but if that doesn't work for you that is okay too. You should be aware though, it is recommended that you stay on a whole diet for at least 30 days before eating anything processed. It is further recommended that you bring back the processed foods one at a time so that you know which foods may cause you issue.

What Is Not Allowed

Just like it is important to know what is allowed when you are eating whole, it is just as important to know what you are not allowed to eat. In fact, this is crucial to your whole food success. Let's say that you find yourself having a craving or you are in a social situation where you do not have access to foods that you know are whole, this is the time when you have a difficult decision to make, and knowing which foods are strictly not allowed will ensure you don't fall too far off of the 'whole' path.

While some items are simply removed during your first month of eating whole (to give your body a true reset), other items are meant to be avoided all the time. It is important to know the difference between these two things and it is even more important that you connect with an experienced whole food eater if you have any questions.

Grains

If you are a whole food meat eater, particularly if you are

following a path like the Whole30, you are essentially eating paleo. This means that you are not allowed to have any grains in any capacity. Here's where it gets a bit tricky, some people are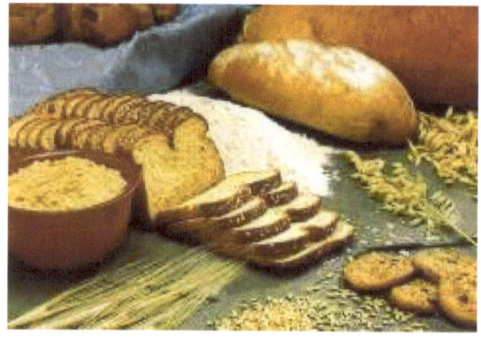

eating whole foods in a more 'Forks Over Knives' sense, meaning they are eating a vegan diet that is typically heavy with grains and legumes.

Despite that though, if you can keep grains out of your system for at least 30 days, when you re-introduce them you will be able to quickly tell if they have a positive or negative impact on your body.

Alcohol

This one could probably go without saying, but it is still worth mentioning. When you consume alcohol, you let a lot of things sneak into your system. But one of the main things about alcohol is that it can be very dehydrating, which will go against the natural digestion process that you are trying to achieve when you are eating whole. It is also a good idea to steer clear of alcohol when cooking.

Dairy

Despite the myths we all grew up with, dairy is not good for your body. There are many reasons for this, but one of the biggest is that dairy is not something that your body can digest easily. Beyond that, many people actually have allergies to dairy and they don't even know it. Things like rosacea and dry cheeks can sometimes be linked to a reaction from dairy.

When you are transitioning into a whole food eating plan, there are some things that you want to be sure to avoid. Eating whole is all about giving your body the gift of true health. But in the beginning, it is also about removing unwanted items from your system. In addition to avoiding the above, you also want to stay away from anything that is processed or contains sugar.

Planning Your Whole Food Meals

If you are new to eating healthy, chances are that you aren't very familiar with the process of planning meals. And this can be extremely intimidating in the first few days, weeks, and even months that you are trying to lose weight.

But over time, this will get easier. You will find that you develop a 'meal planning routine' that will become effortless to you. Over time, you will also learn which meals work best for you and you will add those to your meal schedule for the week.

The most important thing you can do is just get started.

When To Plan

The first thing you should consider when you begin meal planning is when you should actually *plan* your meals. A good idea here is to set aside a designated 'meal planning' date and time and keep it the same every week. This will help you to develop a meal planning routine much faster.

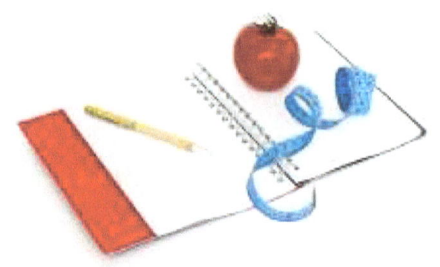

Think about your usual weekly schedule and pick a day of the week when you know you will have some downtime. This should be a time when you won't be interrupted by kids or work and a time when you are the most relaxed. A good example would be a weekend night after the kids go to bed.

What to Plan

Once you decide *when* you want to plan, it is time to think about *what* you want to plan. You want to be prepared for any scenario when it comes to eating. Remember, if you aren't careful just one hunger pain will tempt you to grab the first food that you see. When it comes to eating healthy, being prepared with your meals is essential.

When you sit down to plan your meals, think about what your schedule will be like for the week. Will you be traveling? Will you be going out with friends? These activities will cause you to plan differently than you would if you were due to stay home for the week.

So let's say that you sit down to plan your meals and you realize that you will be traveling this week. What types of things will you want to add into your meal planning because of this? Some easy examples are granola, nuts, and cut up vegetables. You want to look for anything that will last for the car ride and keep you full.

The same principle applies if you are eating out. Think about a few of the possible restaurants you will be going to and figure out what you want to order from each of them. Almost every food chain has their menu and nutritional information posted on their website. This way you will be much less tempted to eat something unhealthy when you get there.

These are just a few examples of what you want to think about when planning your meals and snacks.

Write it Down

Pinterest.com is a good site to find meals made from whole food. Just type in "whole food" (without the quotes) in the Search box. As you find meals that you want to add to your weekly schedule, you will want to write that meal down or save it to your computer to refer to later. But you don't want to stop at simply listing what food you want to eat on what day, you want to list some other key things as well.

First, you want to list where you found the recipe for that meal. Write down the book and page number, website link, etc. so that you can easily come back to it later.

Secondly, you may want to write down the ingredients for each recipe. This will help you to start making your weekly grocery list while you are working on your meal planning.

If you have family members that are not following a whole food lifestyle then you may want to write down their meal plans as well. This is especially useful if you are the one who handles their cooking.

By following these simple planning tips, you will be on your way to whole food weight loss in no time!

Preparing for Weight Loss Success

Many of us have a strong desire to lose weight. Some people decide to start their weight loss journey due to health issues. Other people are looking to increase their energy and feel better overall. And for others, they are looking to lose weight so that they can change their goal weight.

Whatever your reason for wanting to lose weight, there is one thing that is certain...weight loss is hard. It is hard to change the way that you have always been eating. It is hard to eat foods that you might not be a fan of for the sake of being truly healthy, and it is especially hard to lose weight when you are the only one in your circle of family and friends who is trying to lose weight.

There will be bumps in the road. There will be cravings, there will be times when you feel uncomfortable, and there will be times when you are ready to throw in the towel on the whole idea of weight loss. These are natural frustrations when you are following a path that you haven't followed before. And sadly, these frustrations are the main cause for so many people not meeting their weight loss goals. This isn't meant to scare you or make you feel like you can't meet your weight loss goals. This is simply meant to give you an idea of what you can expect.

It is important that you know what to expect, both good and bad, because being prepared for what is to come is the best way to get through these things.

So many times we are told about the good things that happen when you lose weight. And these are great motivators for many people to start their own weight loss journeys. But there is a lot that goes into those weight loss success stories. Believe it or not, every person who has been successful at weight loss has started where you are right now. And most of them have failed at least once before they found success. They didn't know what was ahead but they had a goal in their mind to lose weight no matter what the cost, they made the determination within themselves (mindset) that they were going to lose weight no matter what they needed to do to get there, and many times they had a plan for those times when things got tough.

The same is true for you. If you are reading this you have already made the determination that you are going to lose weight and you have already decided that losing weight is important to you. The only thing you need now is your plan for success. Once you have that, you will finally have everything you need to reach your weight loss goals.

Remember, it doesn't matter where you started from, what matters is where you go from here. If you have stumbled in weight loss before, if you have regained weight, if you have made poor food choices, forgive yourself.

And remember, once you are prepared for weight loss, finding it will be easy.

Choose Your Plan for Success

There is a saying that goes 'if you fail to plan, you plan to fail'. This is true in so many areas of life, but it is especially true when it comes to losing weight. Having a hard time believing it? Here's a simple exercise, think about something that you weren't able to succeed at. Don't think about it with upset or frustration with yourself, rather try to just take an outside perspective of whatever it was that you did not succeed at. Look at some of the areas where you struggled when you were trying to succeed, look at some of the things that you didn't do at the time that you wish you would have done, most importantly look at the areas that you feel had the greatest impact on your inability to succeed.

Would Things Have Been Different If You Had A Plan?

Now let's take a different approach. Look at the situation again, from the very moment that you decided to try to accomplish that goal, and imagine that you had planned for all of the potential pitfalls and successes that you would face on your way to meeting that goal. Do you think having a strategy in place would have changed things for you?

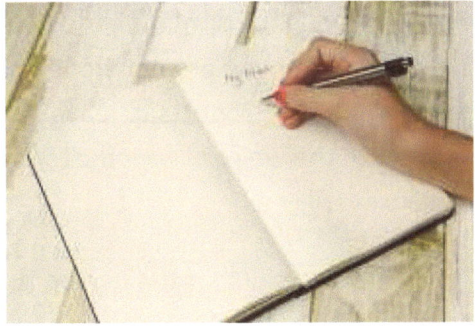

This example isn't meant to make you feel badly about your past decisions, and it certainly isn't meant to make you feel like you did something wrong. Instead, the purpose of this exercise is to allow you to see how valuable it is to have a plan to succeed in place when you start your weight loss journey.

How Do You Find the Plan the is Right for You?

Now that you know how important it is to have a plan, it is time to think about what you need to do in order to create a plan of your own. An important thing to remember here is that a plan that worked for someone else is not necessarily going to work for you. Your plan has to be something that fits into your life and your schedule ... you simply won't succeed otherwise.

Have you ever bought a weight loss or fitness product that came with a calendar and/or meal plan? Has that item led you to your weight loss goal? If it has, then maybe you can tweak it so that you will find even more success using it this time around.

But if the weight loss plan that you bought *didn't* work for you then know that you are not alone. It isn't uncommon for weight loss and fitness products to leave someone disappointed, otherwise the weight loss industry would not bring in billions of dollars every year.

It isn't necessarily that the person that you bought that product from was trying to mislead you, it is simply that the plan that worked for them does not work for you.

Find Clues in the Success of Others

Whether you are trying to accomplish weight loss or another big goal in life, you can find a lot of clues from the people who have walked the path before you. These are people who have already dealt with so many of the things that you will likely be facing and they have been able to overcome these things in order to find success. If you study their journey, you will likely find clues.

So let's say that you a reading an online blog and the writer is talking about the foods that she eats in order to stay full. That could be something that helps you with your own weight loss goals. Before you make this part of your strategy though, you might want to ask yourself:

- Are these foods that I will eat?

- Does this follow with the whole food eating plan that I am on?

- Can I fit these foods into my budget and everyday life?

- Is there any way I can tweak this to fit into my schedule and my life? (for example, ways of preparing the foods, when to eat the foods, etc.)

These are just a few of the things that you might want to consider. You might also want to ask yourself other questions when you look at your weight loss goals. Think about what you want to accomplish and the timeframe you want to accomplish it in. Ask yourself what a legitimate timeframe to reach that goal would be and if you will have any obstacles getting there.

Remember, goals have to be realistic and achievable. Thinking you will lose 30 pounds in two weeks is neither. Those who walked this path before you have a lot of invaluable knowledge to offer. You just need to figure out if that knowledge is useful to you and will help you in your personal journey.

Find Support

Once you have your plan in place your next goal is to find someone to support you on that plan. This can be a coach, a friend, a family member, or even someone you meet online. The goal is to find someone who will be a support system to you when you need it. If you need to go outside of your personal life to find the right support system for you, you can always look at your local health clubs, yoga studios, or health food stores. Because places like these focus on bringing health to the community they will often have workshops, classes, or other fun ways to bring the community together in support of living healthy.

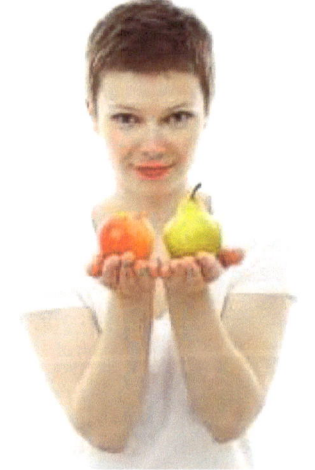

These are just a few of the simple ways that you can begin making your plan for success.

Removing Unhealthy Items

Many times there are things in our home that hinder us from being healthy. Contrary to popular belief, having bad food choices in the home is not the only thing that can keep you from losing weight. If you have items in the home that do not promote a healthy lifestyle, these things can also make it more difficult for you to lose weight.

For example, let's say that you have a pair of skinny jeans that you love, but they don't fit anymore. You don't want to throw them away because they are a reminder of the weight that you once were and they also provide motivation for you to get back to that weight in the future. It might feel like keeping something like this will give you the motivation that you feel that you need, but that might not actually be the case. Many times when we hold onto items like this, they actually don't do us any good. In fact, many times they do the opposite.

Many times keeping something like skinny jeans around the house will make us frustrated with ourselves because they serve as a constant reminder that we are not where we want to be.

And think about all of the people who try to lose weight and then fail to do so, for those people the frustration of not making weight loss work for them will be very hard, and having a constant reminder of how thin they once were might actually make them feel badly about themselves, which could easily trigger them to reach for comfort food.

Because emotional stress can easily make you reach for comfort food, it is also a good idea to get rid of anything that brings back negative memories for you. So let's say that you have a piece of jewelry that you inherited from a relative. While you might love the jewelry, the relative was never very kind to you and often talked about your weight. Even though the jewelry might be pretty, is it really worth it to have something in your home that reminds you of something bad?

Declutter Your Home

Now that you are starting to get rid of things in your home that can trigger a negative emotion for you, it is time to talk about decluttering your home. Many times when we are living in a disorganized home, it can make it harder for us to focus and concentrate. And as you can probably imagine, an environment where you are unable to focus is not the best environment when you are trying to make big changes in your eating habits.

When people think about clutter and weight loss, they often think of it in terms of cleaning out their kitchen. And this is of course very important. But cleaning out the kitchen only solves part of the problem. Granted it is a large part of the problem, but it is not the complete problem.

Having a life that is also free of clutter is the other part of the problem. Being a bit more organized will allow you to think more clearly and plan for your weight loss success more easily.

What To Do With Your Items

Once you have removed everything from your home that stands in the way of your weight loss, it is time to think about what you will do with those items. An important thing to remember here is that even if those items will not work for you anymore, they might still work for someone else. Because of this, it might be a good idea to take your items to a thrift store or hold a garage sale for them.

Preparing yourself for weight loss success isn't just about preparing yourself mentally, and it isn't just about cleaning out your kitchen. Preparing yourself for true weight loss involves getting rid of the things that are holding you back in every aspect of your life.

How to Clean Out Your Kitchen

Now it's time to talk about something that will be a staple in your ability to lose weight, your kitchen. When you have a kitchen that is filled with all of the food items that you are trying to avoid, it can be a huge roadblock in your ability to lose weight. Sure, in the beginning you might have the willpower to stay away from these things, but it won't be so easy when you have been without the foods you love for a few weeks.

If You Don't Need It, Get Rid of It

A good rule of thumb is to get rid of whatever you don't need. You will want to get rid of anything that is processed, filled with sugar, not organic, and dairy.

Grains are a bit different, a whole food eater who is following a vegan (otherwise known as a 'Forks Over Knives' whole food journey will be eating lots of grains. If you fall into this category you will keep your grains and get rid of any meats.

However, if you are following a 'Whole30' type path in your new eating journey, you will be following a diet that is very similar to the paleo diet.

If this is the eating path that you are following, you will want to get rid of all grains, and any meat that is not organic.

What To Do With Your Items

One reason that many people feel uncomfortable cleaning out their kitchen is that they don't like the thought of wasting food.

And that is something that many of us deal with, after all there are so many people in the world that don't have food and it feels wrong to throw out food when so many people don't have it.

If you are trying to determine what to do with your pantry items, it might be a good idea to take them to a food pantry. This is a great way for you to know that the item is going to someone who truly needs it and won't be wasted.

If you have items that can't go to a food pantry, such as opened items or frozen/refrigerated items, it might be a good idea to offer them to a family member or close friend.

What to Do When Your Family Still Eats Differently

One of the most difficult things about changing your eating habits and trying to lose weight is being surrounded by people who are not sharing in your new healthy journey. When these people live with you, the challenge becomes even more difficult. For many people who are trying to eat healthy, the thought of fixing two meals every time they eat, one for them and one for their family, can be difficult. This can be even more difficult after a long day of working and running errands. Luckily there are a few things that may help.

For starters, try to plan all meals in advance. This includes meals that you will be eating as well as meals that they will be eating. Let them know if they want something that is not on their 'meal schedule', then they are responsible for making it. Look for meals that can easily be batch cooked or frozen, this will save you a bit of stress when you are preparing your meals.

Secondly, if your family wants to keep something that you no longer eat, (sweets for example), let them have their own cabinet that you do not have access to. If they want to have cold items in the fridge, it may be a worthwhile investment to get a small second refrigerator to keep your healthy items in.

Organizing Your Kitchen for Whole Food Success

Meal prep can be one of the hardest aspects of adopting a new eating lifestyle. Not only are you changing the things that you are used to eating, which can be hard in itself, but you are likely preparing things that you aren't used to preparing. A great way to eliminate some of the stresses of eating differently is to have an organized kitchen.

Being organized isn't just about knowing where everything is, it is about being able to reach those items quickly. If you have to go digging through cabinets to get the supplies that you need, it will be very hard for you to keep the motivation to make a meal that you have not made before.

Counter Items

The items that you keep on your counter are important for your healthy eating journey. The items you keep on your counter should be the things that you will need to use the most. Generally these are small things, like knives, but they can also be larger appliances, like a mixer. If you are worried about the appearance of clutter on the counter, possibly think about moving some decorations or other items that you don't use on a daily basis.

Cabinet Items

Having an organized cabinet is another area that will save you a lot of time in the kitchen. The lower cabinets are where you will store those larger appliances that you need, but don't use often.

Keep the things that you use the most in the front, the things you use less often a little farther back, and so on. You don't need to get rid of those kitchen items that you love but barely need to use, just keep them in those hard to reach areas of the cabinets, and keep those things that you use frequently in the front.

The higher cabinets are where you will keep your spices, oils, and other non-refrigerated food items. A good rule of thumb here is to keep all spices together, all oils together, etc. If you prep any foods for the week, for example granola, make sure they are kept in an 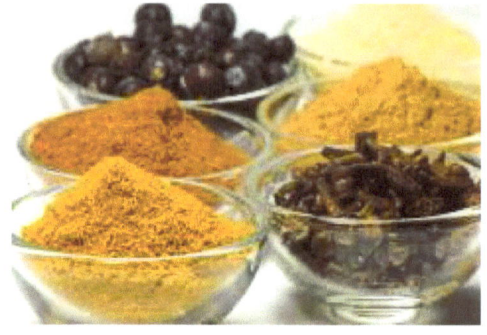 easy to reach place so that you can grab them and go quickly. Sometimes people even opt to keep a list of everything that they have in each cabinet so that they can easily tell what they need more of and where everything is. At first, this might seem like a lot of work, but as time goes on it will get easier.

Using a White Board

A great way to keep yourself organized in the kitchen is to use a white board. Generally people who are trying to lose weight use their whiteboard to track weight loss and food intake, and these are very important. But you can also use your white board to keep your meal schedule, ingredients needed for each meal, and even cooking directions or a shopping list.

Using these simple tips will help you to start losing weight quickly while staying organized in the process.

Other Relevant Books by This Author

If you would like to read more relevant books about this topic, here is a list of the CreateSpace links, titles and descriptions from this author:

https://www.createspace.com/6466393

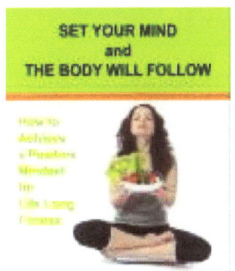

Set Your Mind and the Body Will Follow

The right mindset can completely change your life. That's because it's our mindset that ultimately guides our progress through life and helps us to make the right decisions, including those concerning health and fitness.

It's in your mind that you choose your goals and set course for what you want to accomplish and it's your mindset that allows you to stay focused, stay driven and stay committed until reaching goal.

It's also your mindset that changes the way you present yourself and the way others see you. If you want people to think of you as confident, charming and capable – then you need to project that from within.

Most important of all, it's mindset that allows us to be happy with what we've accomplished and to really enjoy the lifestyle we already have.

By simply shifting your mindset just slightly, you can find health, fitness, contentment, satisfaction and joy in everything you do. You can be more present, more fun and less stressed overnight.

So how on Earth are you going to magically remove the negativity from your lifestyle and create a mindset that the winners of our generation have been working many years to earn.

It's not going to be easy.

You're trying to replicate their years of experience in a much shorter period of time.

But it is possible.

But only if you have someone to guide you. That somebody is me.

I've done exactly this process and I know where the failings are, so I can help you to avoid the pitfalls and thus save time.

Overcome the mental challenges of weight loss. Never again suffer the frustration of yo-yo dieting and eventual weight gain.

https://www.createspace.com/6551526

Change Your Dieting Mindset

Change the way you view "dieting" and never suffer the frustration of yo-yo dieting and weight gain again.

What is the answer to permanent weight loss?

Simple. You need to forget all the incorrect weight loss information you have been given, get off the "diet merry-go round" and learn the healthy weight maintenance formula that will bring permanent and lasting results!

This information works for men or women. And it doesn't matter how young or old you are.

It works even if you have tried to lose weight in the past, and failed.

It works and works well because…

It is NOT temporary
It is NOT restrictive
It is NOT depriving
And it is NOT another "diet"

When you understand the correct formula and what components make up that equation, healthy weight management is within your reach and that is exactly what you get with "Change Your Diet Mindset and Lose Tat Weight Forever".

Get your copy now and stop losing that same 20 pounds over and over!

https://www.createspace.com/6440684

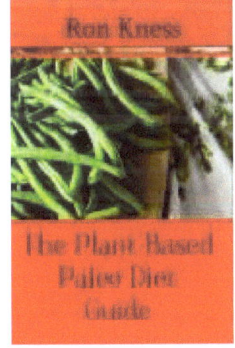

The Plant-Based Paleo Diet Guide

Have you heard about the caveman diet? Also known as the Paleo diet, it mimics the foods that humans ate during the Paleolithic era.

During this prehistoric era, humans ate whatever plants, fruits, vegetables and meats were available to them. That simple nutrition plan means that only natural foods entered their bodies.

Why is that important? Because scientists have studied the remains of humans from the Paleolithic time period, and found they didn't suffer from many of the diseases of today: diabetes, high blood pressure, cholesterol problems, obesity and heart disease.

In short our diet of today is killing us. But you can eat like they did and improve your health. I show you how in this book.

We start out by defining which foods are on and are not on this plant-based diet as a basis to start from. From there we go into some changes that people prescribing to veganism and some vegetarians will have to make to strictly adhere to their choice of eating.

We wrap up with a discussion of meat - the good and bad points, and if you should include it in your Paleo diet or not. After all our ancestors ate quite of bit of meat, but it wasn't commercially farm-raised.

Anyway, I think you will find this book informative and could be just what you are looking for if you are searching for a change from what you are eating now. Enjoy!

About the Author

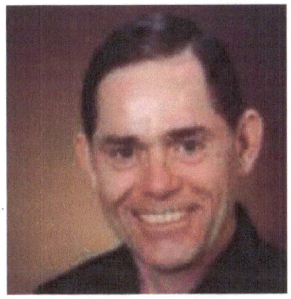

I grew up in Central Minnesota, where my parents owned and operated a fishing resort. Once out of high school I tried a couple of semesters of college, only to quit halfway through the Spring term; I decided at that time that college wasn't for me.

Then I decided to follow my father's previous occupation as an auto mechanic. I graduated from a two-year of vocational training course and worked as a mechanic for five years. While in vocational training, I decided to join the National Guard where I eventually ended up working full-time for 32 years.

So how does all of this relate to writing? In one of my leadership schools, the instructor, who was an English teacher at a juvenile detention center, presented writing to me in a whole new way - a way that started to develop my interest in working with words.

I eventually went back to college on the GI Bill while I was working and earned my Bachelor's degree in Business Administration. Taking a class or two per semester at night and on weekends took me seven years to complete my degree.

Fast forward about 40 years and I now have published over 100 books on Amazon for Kindle, CreateSpace and other publishing platforms.

Besides my own writing, I also ghostwrite ebooks, books, reports, articles, blogs and do Kindle conversions for clients on a variety of topics.

Today my wife and I are retired from our careers and live in Gold Canyon, AZ. I now write as a retirement business where you'll find me happily sitting in my office typing away on my laptop as I work on my next book or ghostwriting project . . . that is if we are not traveling on a cruise ship - our new-found mode of travel.

www.ingramcontent.com/pod-product-compliance
Lightning Source LLC
Chambersburg PA
CBHW050828290526
45792CB00001B/309